BIODYNAMICS OF OSTEOPATHY

Phase Nine

Second Edition

James Jealous D.O.

For more information about Dr. Jealous please visit:
https://BiodynamicsOfOsteopathy.com

BIODYNAMICS OF OSTEOPATHY Phase Nine

Hardback ISBN: 979-8-2955-3932-9
eBook ISBN: 979-8-2955-5621-0

Second Edition 2025

James Jealous D.O. (1943–2021) practiced as an osteopathic physician, teacher and writer for many years. His life's work was to found and develop the specific methodology of Biodynamics of Osteopathy, following the lineage of Dr. A.T. Still and Dr. W.G. Sutherland.

This is one of a series of Biodynamics of Osteopathy books. They grew organically from sets of handouts written by Dr. Jealous and given to students during courses taught by him and his teachers. After many years he collected the handouts together and created individual course manuals, which he added to and rewrote many times. After several more years they evolved further into books.

TABLE OF CONTENTS

OSTEOPATHY IS SERVICE

We use our hands ...

To treat the Whole patient

To listen to the indwelling movements of Life

To treat all levels of illness

To assist in building the patient's functional reserve

To support homeostasis and trophicity by balancing the activity of the autonomic nervous system

To explore "laws not framed by human hands" (Dr. Still and Dr. Sutherland)

To cooperate and communicate with the Laws of Nature (Dr. Wales)

"To find the Health" (Dr. Still)

To get to the treatment plan

To get to the diagnosis

To help establish a point of Rest or Neutral around which the Whole can come to balance

To find Cause

We believe ...

We have an innate capacity to heal

The patient functions as a whole

The autonomic nervous system plays a major role in disease and healing

Structure and function are one form of activity

The Divine is indwelling

Life moves beyond death

There is a Constant Movement toward Normal

We are here to Serve Humanity

Normal is ...

"A sense of peace and harmony" (Dr. Sutherland)

Ease of motion, without tension

A capacity for Neutral

A sense of Wholeness to Life

The capacity for adaptation, change without compensation.

"Skill is proportionate to one's understanding of normal" (Dr. Still)

THIS WORK IS DEDICATED TO RUBY DAY, D.O., MY BELOVED TEACHER AND FRIEND

Her memory rings in my heart. It brings tears of joy, gratitude, and loss to my soul.

She was a real osteopath with a full general practice in the back country of maine when the horse and buggy were still around.

She was disciplined and patient and would not betray will's teaching for the pleasure of power.

She has allowed all of us to grow because she was truly waiting for us without impatience! She kept secrets so well it was easy to believe she had downloaded everything.

I love her sincerely. The longer i am here, the more her directions point me homeward to the cause of osteopathy.

She was a bandito waiting for the gold in each of us. When it arrived, she ignited with fire as she stood smiling with joy.

She lost everything for this teaching ... everything ... and she gained interior peace and nobility with her maker.

She was ahead of her time in every area of health care, from delivery to death.

She was exceptional.

Osteopathy existed before Dr. Still came to it, by suffused contemplation.

You must reach into this source and move freely from it.

There are no authorities in this profession ... none!

There are no teachers, only the eternal nature of the cause of Osteopathy.

AFFERENT HISTORY TAKING AND THE SHAKEDOWN

Rollin Becker D.O. (1964) tells us about afferent diagnostic touch:

> The physician ... has to divorce himself from doing something to the area under examination, thus letting the story come through to him. This is difficult.
> As physicians we are trained to do, and here we are told to let something else do the job of doing ...
> In developing diagnostic touch, there are no "techniques" involved, in the ordinary use of the word.
> The physician lets the innate energies within the health, disease, or traumatic condition of the patient tell the story of the problem involved.
> Thus the physician has no techniques and is in fact told to get out of the way.
> How can the body report if you keep doing something to it during your examination ...
> Be quiet and listen.

THE SHAKEDOWN

The Traditional Osteopathic treatment given by students from the early school through the time I was a student (1965–1970) included a soft tissue treatment that prepared the patient for specific interventions.

The practitioners who used High Velocity Low Amplitude did soft tissue before articulatory techniques to remove compensatory tissue activity and better unveil more primary lesions, as well as build up the energy for treatment of larger lesions.

The Functional Methods did the same but with less force.

Cranial students from William G. Sutherland's study group often went through every segment of the spine, including cranial sutures, looking for and removing as many "trigger points" (called "bowknots" by many) as possible before engaging the Mechanism of Primary Respiration.

This was the basis upon which Will would apply CV4—again, to remove compensatory activity and unveil the primary lesion fields. The refinement of the understanding of the idling or neutral state in the whole patient led to more and more subtle methods, like the CV4/EV4 as we have taught it in earlier phases.

Remember that Power Points also began with this principle, but differently, using a fluctuation of the midline to create a neutral.

The principle involved has not changed and should be honored as much as possible. That is, to bring about as much and as deep and as wholistic an ease in the patient as possible ... reaching toward a complete neutral ... before treatment.

Dr. Day was meticulous about soft tissue, followed by a method to bring the organism to rest as a whole. In other words, to demonstrate a neutral state in the patient as a precursor to treatment.

In 1989, Dr. Becker (a member of the same Sutherland study groups mentioned above) impressed on me "not to start a treatment until the patient's will had surrendered to the will of the Tide" (primary respiration). Again we meet the principle of preparation of the whole patient for a more precise, noninvasive, surgical-like treatment.

Certainly Bill Johnston, D.O., in his Functional Methods, stressed and refined our awareness of neutrality, a state that the practitioner must understand and engage both locally and systemically.

This art is slipping away.

As the years have flowed by full of thousands and thousands of treatments ... I still find it necessary to meet a new patient in a place where they are confident and comfortable with someone's hands on them "doing something." I understand this varies considerably and that a diversity of skills is always on hand to meet the ease of individual persons. However, I have found a method that has the capacity to accommodate almost anyone's needs and allow all of the principles mentioned above to "act."

Many people expect us to manipulate them, and this method can gratify most expectations while leading the physiology toward an ever-deepening neutrality in the whole. This manner of working is a synthesis of all the above methods that I've learned and used separately and in combination for my entire professional life to this very day, now almost fifty years and more than 150,000 treatments later.

This method begins communication between Life, the patient, and the Osteopath, leading in the direction of ease for all three elements.

The foundation of this method lies in one's direct appreciation of what normal is and the changes that occur as *transmutation* moves the system toward a singular and substantial wholeness.

The process appreciates that a resting place, or neutral, is already present, because it has already been established by the Health as a meeting place for wholeness to reside.

One understands that one is not creating neutral but watching the direction of ease in the patient toward a preestablished place.

THE SHAKEDOWN

Practical

The patient is prone ... the feet are off the table so that the talus does not "lock up" and the induced motion does not create a lateral fluctuation.

One is taking more history during the shakedown, the act of which is tempered by the Tide as it suffuses the room in a leading manner. Find the "Tide in the room" and let that level of stillness influence you appropriately.

Begin by moving the tissue and observing the hands migrating around and seeking ease. It feels like playing the piano spontaneously.

Do not move the superficial fascia (work deeply and gently, rocking the whole boat, not vibrating the fluids).

Begin in the paravertebral groove.

The forces placed into the tissue rebound.

The rebound is the source of motion for the next wave.

It will slowly take one into the ease of the whole soma moving around a deep fulcrum.

The rebound is the source of feedback that conditions the action of the observer.

The tissue rebound is elastic at first, then quickly becomes fluid in nature.

At this point there is a clear sensation that one has moved from tissue rebound-moving-tissue to tissue-moving-fluid. The rebound is hydraulic-like. Again, as the fluid forces emerge on the rebound, the tissue on the input changes to a fluid drive and the whole fluid body more or less begins to fluctuate. The physician's intent moves with the quality of the rebound.

Transmutation is occurring.

It eventually settles upon a fulcrum for the whole of Zone B.

Now one clearly sees the Fluid Body suspended upon a fulcrum and being moved through and from the power of that point ... this is quite an event.

Now we "see the point." After a while the fulcrum(s) becomes a midline (reciprocal tension potency only).

A wire appears inside the fluid ... that is, of course, the midline for the fluid in the fluid.

Now we are deep into physiology. The next step is to power point the wire, that is to say, bring the wire down to a Stillpoint by fluctuating it at a pace given by the Tide ... this gentle pumping causes some deep motion toward the center of the whole, as you will witness.

Then the pumping stops just like in the lateral fluctuation, that is to say, the fluctuation becomes self-regulating and our input fades away into a Rising Sea of Silence, where we know that the ship is sailing with the Tide.

Let the patient rest ... Now we have the transparency and simplicity for diagnostics/therapeutics BECAUSE the chaos has been removed and the orderliness of the lesions can be seen and understood.

This is when we begin our diagnostics in a serious case of central nervous system damage.

Discussion

The word "shakedown" originated when a patient coined the term. As the shakedown was progressing, the change in his pocket fell out onto the floor, as it will if you forget, as I did, to have the patient empty their pockets. The patient noticed the change falling out and said, "You're shaking me down," an American term for stealing from someone. I liked his comments and so ... the Shakedown was born.

The interface that extends throughout this treatment is between one's conscience and the natural laws that emerge from the Creator's Hand. The geometry of all motion can be appreciated through the silence from which it sprouts these laws. These motions can move us instead of us trying to move them, and as such, the patient, physician, and Life all move in harmony with the plumb line of creation and the humility of the return to the Health. From this motion one is directed easily and artistically along the pathway created for the return journey that is filled with precision and meaning for the patient. Patients sense this and can easily appreciate that something is being done to correct their dis-ease.

It is very easy to continue the history, which is clarified by the sensory impressions received from the Mechanism and the Health during the journey toward neutral for all aspects of the event.

THE DURATION OF HEALING

Our humanity has the perfect and imperfect juxtaposed in a world of "wills."

Lesions are generally maintained by our imperfect nature, which delays growth.

The cause of this is universally experienced as self-centeredness, the fulcrum of which is so much a part of us that we cannot see it until it disappears for a while.

The pattern of the lesion is spatially and temporally dynamic, living off the energy of Love that has been diverted into a perverse or false fulcrum. Love, being unconditional, does not force one to cooperate ... one is free. Our choices can be hidden, and any attempt to find these hidden pathways cannot be made by that which promotes their activity ... therefore, we need help.

Dr. Becker spoke about Help for an hour one day.

There is help, but we are not aware that being neutral is the only resource we have and that neutrality matures through the help we do not generally notice. Help slips into our world with such ease that we often think we are on a roll and miss the causal relationship of this help.

All motion is animated from one source. If one respects that truth, then discrimination/analysis/conclusions will all fade into a discretion that chooses the Love that is there and clings to that serenity as who one is, as one's identity.

I know that Dr. Sutherland and all my teachers were devoted to being "Centered by the Tide." They knew that struggle was not the primary means of becoming well. This is Osteopathy at work throughout the ages.

"Drink deep, or taste not the Pierian spring." Sutherland begins his text by quoting Alexander Pope ... Why? To express a principle. That is ... Drink from the cup that is given, not your own ... really try to accept this First Principle of Osteopathy ... There is an indwelling capacity to heal BUT not by man-made laws. What a beautiful understanding of life has been given to us.

TRANSMUTATION/REFORMATION

Practical

What I would like you to see is how lesions reform many times during treatment ... this demonstrates how ingrained our self-centeredness is ... the Tide's response to this is Self-Emptying Love ... not a plan formulated to "outsmart the lesion."

We will enter Zone A and a specific lesion field ... treat and watch the Tide transmute the substance, and then watch the substance reform rapidly as the Tide treats it again.

Notice that the Tide will have to keep coming in order to get a real change ... there is a repetitive transmutation/reformation that must create change against the innate nature of the lesion and its subterranean fulcrum.

There is also an attitude in us that thinks the lesion needs to be removed with skill, and this really adds to its "reforming" repeatedly.

ACTION

Humility, that sense of being nothing separate from the Divine Eye Seeing, does not exclude action.

True action is moved from Love and makes our perception exist. We are living effects and as such we can function in harmony with higher principles that take us beyond what we are as self-fulfilling organisms. This Love is self-emptying and by its nature allows us to Serve as part of the Perfect. Perception can be used to Serve something other than ourselves.

We have attempted to enter this balance point between the Perfect and the Disease ... it is a point where the whole of everything is suspended by Love as it works to incarnate the Complete.

In the balance point of everything is The Intention of the Tide and the Liberty to Serve knowingly following the movement of the distortion back to a True relationship with the Blueprint of Life. The guidance for our hands is given by the Seer.

HUMILITY

Humility Is an Aspect of Love.

Humility Is the Effect of a Servant Bonded to the Tide.

One Is Nothing.

This is felt as a reality when one feels the Creator making oneself, as one is being in life.

The sensation of holiness incarnating in what you considered to be your soma is now abiding in Life as a Whole.

Loving the Health in others is a consequence, not an intention.

What God sees exists because the Creator sees it … not because the Creator sees what exists.

The "Dreamer dreaming us" and the "Seer making us" with His Mind blends into a Reality that is Supernaturally suffused with Incarnating Love.

Service is understood as the natural movement of the Intention of the Divine in the Servant.

EVALUATION OF THE CENTRAL NERVOUS SYSTEM

A Biodynamic Summary

Each separate activity is evaluated for the following:

Internal disengagement under the influence of the Tide

Synchronization with the Tide (check for paradoxical motion)

Augmentation with other motions of the system (check for contradictory motions)

Transmutation of the function toward neutral

Activities to evaluate:

The sacs ... (periosteal, dural, brain proper) and the neural tube

Bowing of the tadpole into the Sea around Us

The Tadpole as a whole moving toward lamina terminalis during inhalation (only with rates)

Coiling in the lateral ventricles toward lamina terminalis during the inhalation period

Rocking on the waterbeds

The Bird

Ignition

Motion Present of reciprocal tension potency in the third ventricle central nervous system Fluid Field

Central nervous system collective reciprocal tension potency

Sacral rise with inhalation period; this includes tissue, fluid, and reciprocal tension potency

The effect of Thoracic Respiration on the brain and fluid cisterns

There is a Whole that will appear when the Tide deems it. It is not a vision of all the parts but a transparency that is unlimited and capable of communication. One "sees" via the Seer.

SYNCHRONICITY AND THE CENTRAL NERVOUS SYSTEM

The word "synchronicity" appears in Osteopathy in many contexts. My discussion here is focused on diagnostics, particularly those of the central nervous system and access to the information in the patient.

Dr. Sutherland described involuntary motion in the central nervous system in great detail. "The Tour of the Minnow" is how he chose to create an image for his research. The art of Osteopathy is to observe the natural world and its motion without interfering with Nature.

Sutherland actually said he would teach us to observe without interfering.

Anne Wales writes about synchronization and stillness in the 1953 *OCA Journal.* The Osteopathic ideal is a neutral observer that does not influence the motion being witnessed.

There are many rooms in the cranium. The motion of these rooms should be a Singularity. During inhalation and exhalation, the house should breathe as a whole. This wholeness is rare and, if present, gives one the feeling that there is no anatomy, just a homogenized landscape ... WGS stated, "When all the fulcrums are synchronized, there will be peace and harmony." This state of harmony is so neutral that form is dynamic in its transmutation. Superimposing images (anatomy) on the patient stops intrinsic motion. Following images is also not the highest level of relationship with the Tide.

Ordinarily, we attempt to notice aberrant activity only after we have synchronized with the whole.

These diagnostics relating to synchronicity can take many forms:

1. Asynchrony between the rooms.
2. Paradoxical motion in which the room moves into exhalation during the inhalation phase. This is impossible to notice unless one is synchronized with the motion of the whole house, or better yet, the Tide directly.
3. Contradictory motion between two rooms that are juxtaposed demonstrates opposing physiological motion. Fluid lesions and reciprocal tension potency lesions also occur and will be discussed elsewhere in this course.

Evaluation begins with synchronization with the Tide in the Sea Around Us as it is Now. Do not pick a level of preference. This is our anchor for treatment and diagnostics.

Once we are aware of the Tide, we are centered by it, as Dr. Becker noted. Our task is to feel ourselves being centered by the Tide rather than by our own intention. This discernment is critical. It sets our senses toward Heaven and we see by the Gift of the Tide that we Love. Loving the Tide is the height of innate humility and respect for Life. It is more important than anything one can *do*.

One usually notices the rooms that are fixed and not moving. This is OK but can lead to oversimplification of the patient's needs. Begin as you will, but each room must be seen in detail. This means we must look for motion in the seemingly fixed functions.

Remember that our foremost task here is to be centered by the Tide and then look for motion and the degree of synchronization in each room in response to the breathing of the Whole of Life.

This demonstrates that "Our Skill Is Proportionate to Our Understanding of Normal" ... these words from Dr. Still must be reflected upon very deeply and must be seen directly in this course, in order to follow along with the underlying theme.

Spatial dynamics
Fulcrums
Transmutability
Fluid fluctuations
Reciprocal tension potency dynamic
Power source for Motion Present
Tissue dynamics; that is, the ability to transmute

The key facet of Health is the response of the part to the Whole of the Outside Presence of the Tide.

INVOLUNTARY MOTIONS OF THE CENTRAL NERVOUS SYSTEM

Dr. Sutherland and Dr. Still have pointed us toward the principle of involuntary motion as the foundation of diagnosis and treatment. This essential principle is easily transferred from the hands to the head. Involuntary motion is not an idea. It is a *vital property of life and health.* It is overlooked in most practices. *Involuntary motion is the essence of life* and as such should be in our perceptual agenda as the first question about any dysfunction ... *what kind of motion is present and where?* We must do this service or we will not Think Osteopathy. What is happening ... precisely what details are present in the lesion field, et al., that concern the capacity of the part to function, heal, and express the whole?

Our work here focuses on the central nervous system, but every function must be understood as well as Sutherland understood the central nervous system (see "The Tour of the Minnow"). Our object is accurate diagnosis and the capacity to directly influence the function of the central nervous system once the Tide has done its work ... this will be covered separately as a practical session.

The *inherent motion* of the central nervous system has been a part of Sutherland's teaching for as long as I can recall (since 1966). I will not retrace the steps in his perceptual growth, as we are here in Phase Nine only because we have digested his work in enough depth to bring us to the threshold of a new clinical landscape.

The story can be appreciated from top to bottom or upside down, as the motion is nonlinear and generated for only one moment, then it begins fresh ... it is not repetitive in nature unless the observer makes it so ... each moment there are differences. You can see this in your own life motions as the spirit moves over the waters in you and creates action or work, meaning or skill.

Our first task is to see life moving in what appears as an inconsistent format of movement. *In reality, creation is removing the past so it can find room to incarnate.*

When the observer is nondictatorial, you will see motion unique to the moment ... you will see the transmutational effort and its intention, as well as the method it is using.

Then you decide whether the motion in the central nervous system is coming from an invisible fulcrum that creates another fulcrum for incarnate function and an orderly response in the organism. If so, it is normal ... Our first task is to diagnose the reality of the fulcrum of cause and its incarnate motion present. Or not ... if not, what fulcrum(s) is controlling the function(s)?

If not, is it paradoxical or contradictory?

THE EYE

A healthy eye needs to be irrigated by the River of Life. This Mysterious flow creates all of the physiological events that we reason with, like venous outflow, arterial inflow, and the motion of capillary activity with its intracellular passages. Lymphatic and neurotrophic flow is vital to the homeostatic balance of stress on the eye from a thousand confrontations with glare, dryness, foreign bodies, infectious agents, genetic liabilities like glaucoma and macular degeneration and all the diseases that enter a family practice doorway.

Healing often depends on involuntary motions like those described above, plus the few we understand from observing the magical Tidal motions of Thoracic and Primary Respiration.

What we may not think about when we Think Osteopathy and indwelling physiology is the spatial dynamics of normal flow, that is to say, the interconnectedness of all the apparent individual flows in a universal movement in the whole, which forms the parts.

This is our goal, to see the whole alive and well ... *to see the parts means there is a lesion ... this alerts us to treat the eye as a whole and reevaluate the parts until they are barely visible.*

The optic chiasm is a fulcrum that is inside the Lamina Terminalis. It should, like any fulcrum, shift. As the eyes move, they augment the motion of the whole central nervous system. That is to say, during the inhalation phase the globes and all functions move toward the Lamina Terminalis, and the shape changes to be shorter and fatter, as does the whole organism. This motion of the globes and the boney orbits are thusly synchronized and easily evaluated. The general posture of the eyes can be myopic or hyperopic depending on whether they are locked in the inhalation or exhalation posture.

INVOLUNTARY MOTION

Practical

Where's the fulcrum for the following?
The optic axis
The cause of the spatial dynamics now and in the beginning

Motion present in ...
Orbit as a shape ... fulcrum
Globe as a shape ... fulcrum
Neurotrophic flow via the optic nerve
Internal physiological augmentation
Present fulcrum for the whole
Health: the original fulcrum of cause

Treatment method:
Wait and watch—with neutral senses.

FIRE

We have begun to see potency as a reality rather than an idea.

The reality of the mystery of potency was mentioned hundreds of times by Dr. Sutherland.

His experience of this potency, or power, was that it was potent beyond any scientific explanation yet discovered.

This potency was often held in a Mysterious silence, both literally and figuratively. Often beginners were not allowed to even know about it. In 1992 I actually witnessed anger by a teacher because a table trainer mentioned the word ... this kind of elitism is now dying away due to the respect that a community generates within itself. *Respect for what we do not know is the foundation of a living relationship with the Tide.* This is a phase of humility rather than elitism.

Potency is not a descriptive term.

Often when we see the therapeutic forces at work, we see Fire doing the work we ascribe to the potency. In my experience, when we teach fire as the substance that is breathing in and out rather than a mechanical shift, students come to a realization that the *Potency of the Tide* is a transmutative force of astounding proportions. This changes the idea of the potency into an appreciation of it as a *living flame*, an aspect of the Breath of Life that can consume a lesion field relative to its neutrality.

The writing of the Christian mystic Dionysius (below) is so clear. His description shows that he saw inside the nature of the Fire rather than just looking from the periphery at phenomena ... His observer was part of the Fire, not separate from it.

This is the point of our work in this practical session: seeing inside the Nature of Fire and its effect on the senses.

I believe that working with the fire in a seam can be particularly enlightening, but any manner of engagement is valid.

Let's choose a seam that is relative to the patient's needs and give a real treatment.

Observe Fire, let your eyes see inside the Flame.
Fire is in all things
Is spread everywhere
Pervades all things without intermingling with them
Shining by its very nature, hidden
Manifesting its presence only when it can find material to work on
Violent and invisible
Having absolute rule over all things
It comprehends but remains incomprehensible
Never in need
Mysteriously increasing itself
Showing forth the nature of its Majesty, according to the nature of the substance receiving it
Powerful and Mighty
Invisibly present in all things

Dionysius, Christian Mystic
(AD 20–90)

REVIEW OF CREATION COMMENTARIES

The spoken word from the Divine passes through the watery substance of the silence and creates the ground from which life sprouts. This process is never-ending. All life becomes and is renewed from this constant flow.

One can see this happening as the love returns from the inner matrix of one's being (soul) to the Creator.

Inherent motion is present before any form is visible to the outer senses. *Imagine an invisible design that precedes the known and does not develop as the parts grow but is complete at conception.*

This event is free from genetic influence ... to know this, one discerns the truth in oneself and the man-made tendencies that are ethnocentric.

Sutherland stated that the formative and the restorative forces have an unerring power. The cause of the accuracy and intelligence of these forces is a mystery that can be engaged but not dissected.

The embryologist DeHaan states that the power of growth never misses a geometric intersection—another illustration of the perfect matrix present as Cause.

All of this becomes visible in the right light.

THE BIODYNAMIC MODEL

When we begin, we generally are fixed on anatomy. As our senses loosen, we see forms and patterns of moving tissue ... the static fades, and with that our thinking changes.

Once involuntary tissue motion is easily witnessed, one is at the edge of the transmutative process, where physiology is in the foreground, comingled with fluid dynamics.

One has entered both the form and function of a living system ... it becomes obvious that any division of life into structure and function is naive at best. Again our thinking must change to include form, function, and transmutation as a kaleidoscopic puree dancing, dying, and reforming in a new species. Remember, we are alive, all of us!

When we move on, we enter Silence, Stillness, and Space. This nothingness is frightening. Its Presence causes many to drift sideways for a while, protecting their possessions. Unknowingly, the traveler gets faith and momentum when these possessions become the raw substance of a dynamic transmutation of the soul; the senses enter into darkness. In the darkness one finds Life and Creation.

The movement of a refined and Holy Silence pours into our awareness. From the substance that is poured out of the Silence comes the ground from which all inherent functions arise and receive their Nurture.

The whole process of Life is nothing like any book you will ever read ... it is unlike any thought you can imagine, because nothing lasts more than a few seconds in the crucible.

From *Autobiography of Andrew Taylor Still*:
"As an electrician controls electric currents,
so an Osteopath controls life currents
and revives suspended forces.
To turn on the blaze of an incandescent light ..."

THE MARK OF CREATION

The Scripture of the Tide Washes Ashore, Leaving Traces in the Sands of Time.

Jacques Duval, D.O., of Paris, France, was a great Osteopath. He taught and wrote for forty years or more and was one of the early few to see that the formative forces of the embryo were present in the adult. He loved me very deeply and I found him to be an Oasis for me. His friendship with Rollin Becker extended over a lifetime, and Jacques was often here in the United States with us all.

In his office, hanging in the waiting room, there were two sentences:

"Les enfants sont nes de la lumière, et ils sont porteurs de la lumière."

"Et si cette lumière a été voilée par quelque obstacle, le rôle de l'ostéopathe est de savoir écarter cet obstacle, et comme dit Rollin Becker, de recréer la lumière."

Translation:

"Children are born of light, and they are carriers of light."

"And if this light has been veiled by some obstacle, the role of the Osteopath is to know how to remove this obstacle and, as Rollin Becker says, to recreate the light."

At my request, this information was retrieved by Mark Barker,

D.O., of Paris, a longtime dedicated student of Jacques's. I had seen it in Jacques's office and was curious. I was told that the first sentence was a quote from Walter Russell. After Jacques died, I believe his belongings would have been destroyed. Many thanks to Mark, who overcame the obstacles and took Jacques's papers into safekeeping.

NATURAL BOUNDARIES

Treating can be deeply fatiguing; this is because we do not see the Intention of the Tide.

Why? There are many reasons, all of which are beliefs, fears, or habits. Some of the habits develop from the deafness of our culture and two-dimensional education.

An overview of the natural progression in the development of skill may be useful. We begin by learning the efferent art of palpation. We search the patient's body for lesions; once they are found, we come to a conclusion and apply forces along the "tracks" created by our diagnostic method. Forces are applied in varying degrees and then reevaluation helps us prognosticate.

The output from the clinician is considerable, but there is also fatigue and boredom in the soul caused by repetition. Defining our relationship with Nature through mechanical forces competes with the movement of Creation; one tires from all of this. The usual outcome is authoritative behavior.

This begins the art of Osteopathy in most schools.

As we adjust to being in the physiology instead of the anatomy, we enter the world of involuntary motion. The boundary between the tissue and the fluid fades as one becomes more docile and afferent, listening to motion rather than inertia. One begins to enter the world of sensing, and even the history from the patient flows more easily. Now one adds balanced membranous tension.

At first one cannot help going into barrier due to mental habits, but eventually (after years) the point of balance and the balance point emerge as precursors to the entry of the Physician within the patient as force or potency that does not act mechanically. This functional approach is a major shift because the direction of ease remains as a constant pathway to neutral in the whole and a dependency on indwelling therapeutic forces. This is the passage from theoretical Osteopathy to direct awareness of natural laws or principles at work in us all. At this level of work, many years pass as one refines the relationship expressed by the Balance Point, the Point of Balance, Stillness, Pauses, Neutrals, and unconditional or unpredictable activity, all of which must be Trusted in order for one to live more deeply in the "waters of Life."

As long as we add any force or desire to help, we lose vital force from within ourselves and do not become refreshed easily. We become aware of what leaves us and what comes into us during an office visit. This knowledge makes us aware of natural boundaries innate and indwelling in us since conception.

As time passes, one begins to look for the blueprint or intention of the healing forces. One begins to observe the Health and the interface between disproportion and the generative forces that align one with the Singular Fulcrum of the Original Matrix. As we work to understand, we get very tired analyzing and changing habits. Patience is an indwelling function of neutrality, but one tends to try to be something that is already invisibly present and coming into view. When one starts seeing the innate and the natural boundaries, the fatigue lessens. Joy arises for no apparent reason. We have stopped leaning into life in order to comprehend and participate ... strangely, the Joy increases, as does the quality of one's listening and interest in others as Self.

Let Life flow, and watch. Withdraw your output and let the Great Tide sweep you upward and into the company of Wisdom. Be still ... still ... really peacefully indifferent, and you will find that Osteopathy exists without your personal energy.

Practical

During this course we hope to find a balance point in the interface between the pattern of disease and the Perfect Health. Once the balance point comes into your awareness and All function is suspended... Then slip the reciprocal tension potency in the lesion field onto the perfect template. This is done with NO resistance from the Tide that is holding our awareness inside of Itself. It takes a little time and is ONLY used as fine-tuning.

Once the lesion is on center, withdraw your attention.

As you will recall, Sutherland did fine-tuning only when the system had fully demonstrated the capacity for change and healing was already in progress.

This is direct action done by the Tide ... it may sound like you are doing something, but read the steps carefully, as no force will leave you and no isolated decision will occur. The balance point is in the whole of the therapeutic reserve.

NEUTRAL AND REGENERATION

"When matter ceases to be divisible, it then becomes a fluid of life

and easily unites with other atoms and is a mass or body of living matter and recrystallizes into the form given by the parent causes."

From chapter XI of A. T. Still's The Philosophy and Mechanical Principles of Osteopathy, 1892, p. 254–255

In the most minute particle of bioplasm there is a center of vitality. To this center nutrient matter comes from the circumference to be vitalized and to enter the cycle of perpetual movement from center to circumference.
New matter is formed in these vital centers. ... A complex process goes on, (a) bioplasm selects the nutrient matter from the blood, (b) the blood in turn is tissue and as such is formed by bioplasmic processes. ... The vital action in all cases is at some center of bioplasmic mobility. ...
This center of life receives its illustration embryologically in connection with the nucleus of the fecundated ovum, the primary origin of vitality in the newly formed organism. ... this already existing bioplasm in the centers of life renders possible the physical and mechanical phenomena, which we call change of matter. The bioplasm thus possesses a vital force which it can project into the non-living, drawing it

closer to its center of life, then projecting it outwards toward the circumference of tissue and organ formation.

Dr. J. Martin Littlejohn, Ph.D., M.D., D.O., L.L.D., First Dean of the College of Osteopathy, Kirksville Missouri; founder of the Chicago College of Osteopathy; and founder of the British School of Osteopathy.

The Journal for the Science of Osteopathy, Vol. 3, No. 4, August 1902.

OSTEOPATHY

"When a century later historians are sifting the events of this time for the epoch-marking discoveries of science and civilization, there will be few chapters more important, I think, than that devoted to the reformation in medicine which will have come about through the acceptance and practice of Dr. Still's system known as Osteopathy."

Robert L. Taylor (1850–1912)
He served as the governor of Tennessee from 1887 to 1891 and from 1897 to 1899. He also served as a United States senator from 1907 until his death in 1912.

From the 1906 *Journal of the American Osteopathic Association*, Vol. 6, p. 11

IF

If you sense a Living patient under your hands and if you sense the Health first and if you synchronize with Beauty before the Lesion and if you are a true scientist without bias and if you Listen instead of Speak with your hands and if you can wait for your mind to be Neutral and if you are not distracted by former skills and if you are not trying to fix only the Symptoms and if you can see the direction of ease and if you understand Dr. Still's first chapter in *Philosophy of Osteopathy* and if you believe that your hands can show you more than you can show them and if you believe that your job is to follow and not to lead the Mechanism of Life and if you can look for something new in each treatment and if you are trying to cooperate with Laws not framed by human hands and if you believe that Life is Eternal and if you burn all the books once you have a foundation and if you can enter the wilderness inside yourself and the patient and if you believe Love is the Cause of everything and if you can take opposition without resistance and if your mind wants to be Transparent to your own Health and if your Ignorance does not hide but becomes humble and if you see all forms of Osteopathy as branches on one tree and if you have read Sutherland again and again and again and if you see that Thoracic Respiration Neutrals are a priori to a Complete Neutral and if you know that there is no form without formlessness and no Life without Death, Transmutation, and Renewal, and if you know that the treatment is already waiting in the patient and if you know that your help is what is needed for a hundred reasons and if you know we only help the treatment begin and if you know that it is self- sustaining and if you can love people who destroy the treatment before they leave the office and if you do not expect more from yourself than what God grants you and if you know you must leave everything you know behind in the dust of yesterday and if you know stillness is not Stillness and if you teach only from what you love and if you can be fearlessly Neutral in your heart and breathe, and if you can feel the Health when you cannot feel it … THEN, my friend, you will be a Joyful Beginner Osteopath. Then, if you wish, your prayers will be answered.

GREECE IS WHERE MUCH OF OUR LANGUAGE ORIGINATES

The "cause" of a word is an attempt by a human being to communicate a relationship that already exists. When a human being is able to sit near the River of Life and be impartial to the senses, he or she is awakened by the senses to the world of Cause. One could easily say that genuine words are born out of a silent relationship between man and the Creator.

A friend of mine studies ancient Greek. Below is an example of how a word flows into being:

Doctor comes from iatros.

Iatros has as its root iaomai, which means to treat or heal.

Iaomai has its cause in "ia" which means sunbeams or arrow-like rays.

What is your sense of these roots?

THE TIDE EBBS

The Tide ebbs

But always comes in again.

Bend to the oars

Secure the balance point

And allow the tide to carry on

To the osseous shoreline borders

W. G. Sutherland, D.O.
Advanced course, 1949

PERCEPTUAL STUDIES – THE FLOW OF THE ATTENTION

Motion is the essence of Life.
Where there is motion there is a natural flow of Neutrality and Wholeness.
Voluntary motion is controlled by the attention of the individual.
Involuntary motion is the expression of wholeness.
Involuntary motion is the essence of Osteopathy.
The flow of attention from the Seer creates the seen and the unseen.

***

Our attention can be quite fixed, that is, it lacks motion.
The state of our attention conditions what we perceive.
It also has a tremendous effect on our sense of wellness.
Stasis precedes disease.
Both disease and pain are related to static attention.

Education trains the attention to converge, to go to a place and hold there, stopping the natural flow and creating a separation from the Health. The result is loneliness and grief, often unseen, but lurking in the subconscious.

Normal attention flows like warm honey.

When it flows, it's moved by the Health toward its cause.

We can study the flow/stasis of attention and observe the movement of the attention when it is free and flowing. This task requires mental concentration.

THE STUDY OF THE ACTIVITY OF ATTENTION

"Our Skill Is Proportionate to Our Understanding of Normal"

Dr. Still's words will challenge us *not to look at our capacity to find lesions* but to understand normal physiological motions. This knowledge is not in books. One must see normal by the power of observation.

What is the normal movement of attention?

We begin our study by watching our attention ...

Is it focused and fixed on a place?

Where is the fulcrum that controls the attention?

What is the cause of the act of the attention?

Is it flowing from inside to outside ... freely ... fixed ... where does it originate? All this we do by sensing the attention as it works or as it locks up and lesions (stops flowing).

Let it flow to the interior of yourself. What does it do? Where does it flow? Does it stop on a thought or a feeling? Does it flow into a place?

As the day passes, every once in a while, try to see what your attention is doing and record the event ... remember, we are trying to understand normal, that is, what does the attention do when allowed to express its Truth, its Motion.

The attention is a substance, an energy that flows from the Source of Life and as such is naturally at work following the intention of the Breath of Life.

When the attention is free to move, one does not feel time or death or separation from anything, even enemies.

Ruby Day talked about attention as force. She said that Sutherland taught that it was more than enough force to add to a treatment when using midline dynamics. She trained me to know when to use the attention as a tool and when to literally withdraw it, so it was not an inhibitory force.

The attention was never fixed for more than seconds and only in an attempt to ignite the reciprocal tension potency and set it in therapeutic motion, similar to a lateral fluctuation.

When someone fixes their attention too long, it is not only uncomfortable for the patient but also can lesion living substances. The attention and the intention should flow through everything and not be directed by us.... The flow of Wisdom will do work that will organize everything into the flow of normal.

A neutral mind has no personal intention. It is impartial, lacks partiality to all things or outcomes, thus allowing the automatic shifting of one's perception by the River of Life.

Convergent and divergent language are discussed in Ken Robinson's YouTube videos on the subject; Drs. Sutherland and Still stressed divergent thinking as the means of exploration into "laws not framed by human hands."

During treatment, the attention should be moved by the Tide, not by our intention.

THE TIDE

William Garner Sutherland gave a speech to the Rhode Island Study Group on May 10, 1949. Here is a quote from it.

> The breath of air is a material. But the Breath of Life is something we cannot see ...
> ... something invisible, a Potency. ... a potent fluctuation, something that is Intelligent ...
> I'm referring to the Breath of Life in that Tide, the fundamental principle in the Primary Respiratory Mechanism.
> The Breath of Life, the highest known element to which Dr. Still called your attention. ...
> That's what I want you to see, the potency in the fluctuation of the cerebral spinal fluid, and most of all ... the Breath of Life ...
> ... that spiral movement on the slow movement of the Tide ...
> Let's call this whole unit here in the audience the Tide. It's all the same cerebral spinal fluid. It all has the Breath of Life. ...
> You notice that change in the Tide ... this room? ...
> It's bringing you close to something that Dr. Still realized, the closeness of his maker ...
> ... the Intelligence of that fluid ... Something that nourishes nerve cells, The Breath of Life. ...
> We're getting back to Dr. Still's science of Osteopathy ... It's the truth. It can never die.

BIODYNAMICS OF OSTEOPATHY BOOK SERIES

This book is one of a series of twelve *Biodynamics of Osteopathy* books. It is recommended that you read the whole series in order, as each book builds on the understanding from prior books. It is also recommended that you seek experienced teachers and mentors to help you experience the full depth of the information given.

The full series is as follows:

Phase One is about involuntary motion, which is motion present in the whole and in the lesion. We learn to synchronize with the breathing of Primary Respiration before we approach any treatment. This synchronization is the key to working with stable rates and not irritating the system. The principle of synchronizing with a healthy aspect of the patient suffuses the whole teaching program. This synchronization shifts our awareness to a different level of receptivity, which allows us to see Primary Respiration rather than the lesion field, and this eventually leads us to an understanding of the intention of Primary Respiration.

Phase Two is about communication with the natural laws of healing that surround activity at 2 to 3 cycles per minute. We synchronize with the breathing of Primary Respiration and also add the skill of sensing the fulcrum, the Stillness through which the breathing creates form and function. It is a different kind of synchronization from that in Phase One, shifting our awareness more deeply. As this occurs, the treatment automatically expresses itself. The end point of treatment, when compared with Phase One, reveals several differences. We find this kind of synchronization works exclusively with the fluid body and the outcome of treatment is more complete than when working with tissue alone.

Phase Three is centered around the activities of the Long Tide (100 second cycle). We explore an indwelling therapeutic force already present in the lesion field. We learn that the dural system is not made-up of three sickles but rather a series of folds in a sac, arising during growth and development. We see the relationship between the upper and lower dural sacs, awakening us to the independence of two separate tentorium cerebelli. We discover that zone D, the horizon, and the Wire (along which the Long Tide moves during its intended therapeutic course) are all linked as natural laws pertaining to this level of Primary Respiration.

Phase Four focuses on the Midline, a place where the spatial relationships are expressed as a whole. It synchronizes and centers us in such a way that we become aware of Zone D and the Dynamic Stillness. The Third Level Stillness in Phase Four is different from the Stillness in the other Phases – we are centered by the Stillness at the center of creation. Our intention is replaced by the intention of the Tide which can facilitate our spiritual path.

Phase Five is about *the face*. As we approach the face, we use all of the principles that we have learned in Phase One, Two, Three, and Four. We work with automatic shifting and notice differences from how the face is viewed by older models within Osteopathy in the Cranial Field. As we synchronize with the therapeutic presence of the Long Tide we see what we can learn about the face from that landscape. We also work with Seams, Dynamic Stillness, and Ignition.

Phase Six is a continuation of our journey into the Wholeness that generates life and delivers therapeutic forces that transmute lesions once Neutral is expressed. It is a mixture of activities centered around the outside presence of Primary Respiration as something that is a non-biological force and that has a persona. We will also continue to explore seams and then move on to the extremities, first in the embryological terms and then as Sutherland taught them in his work called PowerPoints. Phase 6 is a time to build your understanding of the Tide and refine your skills.

Phase Seven highlights the Health. Dr. Still's famous comment "Find the Health; anyone can find disease," has plagued many minds over the last century. We come to the clear vision of several indwelling aspects of the Health: Love ... liquid light ... and a diamond matrix. A approach to the terminally ill and dying patient is addressed. In the somatic sensation of the Tide passing through the House Under the Sea, our awareness is transmuted by the Health. The lesion is seen as a precognitive act of the Health. Thoracic Respiration, Primary Respiration, and Ignition are as One. The landscape is vast ... and the principles of healing are even more substantial than we have previously experienced.

Phase Eight is a deeper exploration of seams, balanced rhythmic interchange, and the Flame of Intention as a therapeutic modality. Phase Eight is the culmination of our awareness of Wholeness, and ultimately brings us to the Divine Presence, Unconditional Love and Oneness. The living Tide dominates the awareness while forms move to the background. One feels the Breath of Creation in oneself as the Center of Wholeness. One feels the Unfoldment of oneself as one is Created. Our consciousness is a gift; we do not own it and if we try to control it we lose Wholeness.

Phase Nine is when we are able to fully evaluate and treat the Central Nervous System and the Eye. We also address Fire and the therapeutic modality of the Shakedown. True action is moved from Love and makes our perception exist. This Love is self-emptying and by its nature allows us to Serve as part of the Perfect. Perception can be used to Serve something other than ourselves. We have attempted to enter this balance point between the Perfect and the Disease ... it is a point where the whole of everything is suspended by Love as it works to incarnate the Complete. In the balance point of everything is The Intention of the Tide following the movement of the distortion back to a True relationship with the Blueprint of Life.

Pediatrics One explores how children grow as a whole, not in parts as we sometimes believe. Children live in the Direction of Ease of motion present in their fluid metabolic fields, otherwise they get uncomfortable and require assistance. Does your treatment directly support the whole, or does it assume to support the whole? We realize children are not adults and cannot be treated as adults are. We approach the therapeutic modality of the "Meeting Place", prenatal and postnatal periods, the treatment of the pelvis during pregnancy, fetal malposition and labor.

Pediatrics Two is where we deepen in the perceptive awareness necessary to approach the treatment of children. We deepen in our appreciation of Wholeness, the three levels of Stillness and the "Meeting Place". We approach "Desert Neutral", where therapeutics pass into the neutral substance, and a mystery unfolds as the breath of Divine love cascades as a therapeutic force across a night desert landscape, filling and leaving behind no visible effects. We further address treatment of the pelvis and the uterus during pregnancy. We explore thoracic and Primary Respiration in children, and the Family Circle.

Pediatrics Three is where we continue to study the therapeutic Flow of Attention. We deepen in Third Level Stillness and the Meeting Place. The Meeting Place is easily misinterpreted ... our observer must be so still and neutral that the process can be seen as it happens. The central nervous system in the child can be finally approached for evaluation and treatment. We explore teething and also the "locked up head". We use the therapeutic modality of the Flame of Intention, and its connection to the Breath of Life. Everything is transparent to the Breath of Life.

ABOUT THE AUTHOR

James Jealous, D.O. (1943–2021), was an osteopathic physician, teacher, and writer. His life's work was founding and developing **Biodynamics of Osteopathy**, a unique methodology he established within the field of osteopathy, following the lineage of Dr. A.T. Still and Dr. W.G. Sutherland.

He was born in Saco, Maine, and since his father was an osteopathic physician, he was around osteopathy from an early age. He studied at Kirksville College of Osteopathic Medicine in Missouri (now the A.T. Still University of Health Sciences), graduating in 1970. He then set up practice in rural Maine as an osteopathic primary care physician.

Over time, Dr. Jealous saw parallels between the work of embryologist Dr. Erich Blechschmidt and that of osteopathic physician Dr. William Garner Sutherland. This inspiration led him to create his own body of work. In the early 1990s, he began teaching "A Biodynamic View of Osteopathy in the Cranial Field," which, as he developed his specific methodology, was refined to "Biodynamics of Osteopathy."

A deeply spiritual person, he felt most at home in the natural world and was an avid fisherman and hiker.

For more information, please visit:
https://BiodynamicsOfOsteopathy.com

There is a wind passing through …
it is the motion of creation,
the eternal motion of Divine love.